Hotlifestyle

Sweet dreams are made of this.

Sleep Strategies

PAUL McQUEEN

Graystone LA
Tanner Business Centre
Chew Valley Road
Oldham OL3 7NH
United Kingdom

www.hotlifestyle.info

First Edition

Medical Disclaimer: This book is not intended as a substitute for medical advice from a physician. It contains information that is intended to help readers be better informed consumers of health products and activities. Any use of this information is at your own risk. Before beginning any new physical activity or changing calorie intake, it is recommended that you seek medical advice from your doctor. The information provided in this book is for general informational purposes only.

WHAT OTHERS ARE SAYING

„In today's high-octane, high-pressure world, Paul's new book is like a welcome island in turbulent seas. Everyone loves a self-help book. But we often rush our fences in trying to make every change at once. Paul guides us through making sustainable and effective steps towards a more enjoyable life on every level. Highly recommended."
Claire Meadows - Editor in Chief, After Nyne Magazine, and former Huffington Post blogger

„From managing stress and anxiety to the art of good communication, finding your true vocation and improving sexual intimacy, McQueen writes with great insight and relevance - supported by highly effective techniques, exercises and personal challenges that will help create positive and lasting changes to our health, wealth, relationships and much more."
Martin Gill - Assistant Editor, Yoga Magazine

„Paul McQueen has written the ultimate self-help book. Comprehensive and accessible, Hotlifestyle is a lifestyle, not a book. It covers all aspects of life with great summaries of each chapter. This brilliant book gives you the tools to make great choices and live your best life. Life-changing stuff."
Catherine Balavage - Editor, Founder and Publisher, Frost Magazine

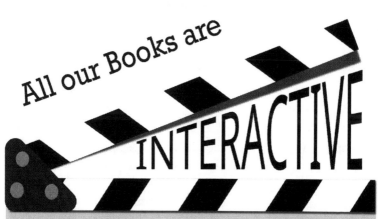

All our Books are INTERACTIVE

Free Online Bonus Material

Step 1
Scan the QR

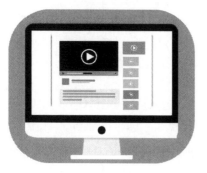

Step 2
Watch the Videos

GET THE MOST OUT OF THIS BOOK

Getting a good nights' sleep requires taking a critical look at the reasons why you can't sleep, understanding the mechanics of sleep then creating an effective routine to improve both quality and quantity. No matter how much it impacts your life right now, implementing some easy to follow techniques and making the necessary changes will improve your situation.

In your enthusiasm to get cracking you might be tempted to read this book from cover to cover without acting on it. Take your time, it's not a race.

Each chapter conveys the latest evidence-based findings, written in a concise, no nonsense format. Read each chapter through so you understand the bigger picture. Go back and work on the parts you think will benefit you the most. Finish each section before going on to the next. You might not need to take any action from some chapters, but read them anyway, remember, knowledge is power.

Exclusive to this book are links to hotlifestyle.info that take you deeper into the subject matter. The level of success you achieve comes down to the choices you make after reading this book. What you choose to focus on during the next few weeks will decide what level of success you will achieve during the next few months. Are you ready to lay down some sleep strategies?

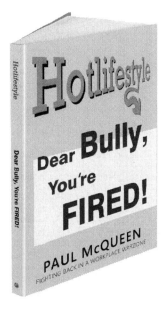

Dear Bully, You're Fired!

The best course of action to get rid of your bully, once and for all.

With a pull no punches approach Paul McQueen takes you on a journey of realization offering real answers showing you a step by step plan to getting your bully fired. You decide whether to play softball or hardball with the bully. He will help you align your emotions to cope with the darn awful situation you find yourself in changing your whole way of thinking.

With your livelihood and sanity on the line the stakes are high. Give yourself a fighting chance to stop them in their tracks by understanding that bullies won't engage where they can't easily win.

Bullying in the workplace will only get worse as pay increases and promotions become more scarce creating a cutthroat behavior as people battle for position in the company food chain.

One day, simply by placing this book with its 128 pages of ground breaking advice in full view on your desk, will stop bullying in its tracks.

GETTING TO SLEEP

THE MECHANICS OF SLEEP

SLEEP STRATEGIES

TIME FOR A WAKE-UP CALL

ANXIETY AND SLEEP

STRESS AND SLEEP

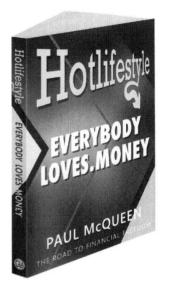

Everybody Loves Money
ISBN 978-1-9164969-9-6

The Best Handbook for Dealing with Money Matters

Packed with practical, actionable tips to lift your personal finances up to the next level. Take back control, keep a grasp on your hard-earned cash and start working towards financial independence.

www.EverybodyLovesMoney.com

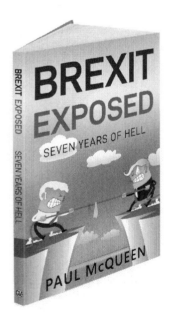

Brexit Exposed
ISBN 978-1-9164969-4-1

Seven Years of Hell

Read about a time when the UK Parliament defied their voters, trying to stop Brexit from ever happening by any means. Who lied, who predicted the end game and who made a fool of themselves.

www.Brexit.Exposed

INTRODUCTION

Imagine how different your life would be if only you could get a good nights' sleep.

I'm sure you consider those who easily fall asleep as simply the lucky ones. Some go through life never having to consider sleep at all, some of us are going to have to work at it on a night by night basis. Yes, getting your just deserved shuteye takes some work, but it may be the most rewarding you will ever do.

There has been real progress in recent years in understanding how to achieve a good nights' sleep. It's sometimes about the lifestyle choices you make and the ability to practise good long-term habits, keeping an open mind when it comes to change.

You certainly don't need me to tell you that we live in a 24/7 society in which sleep deprivation has become the norm. Most of us aren't getting enough, and the all-too common attitude of 'Plenty of time for sleeping when I'm dead' might just bring it closer, death that is.

We are experiencing a sleep crisis. The Centers for Disease Control and Prevention (CDC - US government organization based in Atlanta) declared insufficient sleep as a public health epidemic back in 2011, and the situation has become worse.

Recent research has shown that nearly 75% of those surveyed said they slept less than seven hours per night; 12% got less than five hours a night; 30% complained of ‚poor sleep' most nights - with the top three reasons being stress and anxiety (45%), partner disturbance (25%), and general noise (20%); while more than one in 10 cited having an uncomfortable bed.

Scientists agree that quantity and quality of sleep impacts how we look, determines our mood and performance, and influences practically every facet of our life.

A Stanford University study showed that people who had five hours or less sleep a night had 15% more of the hormone ghrelin (which stimulates appetite) and 15% less of the hormone leptin (which lets you know you are full) than people who slept for eight hours. So, sleep more and you'll want to eat less; that's the best weight loss technique I've ever heard of!

What has sleep got to do with living a Hotlifestyle? Realizing that a Hotlifestyle is relative to your current standpoint is the first step to a deeper understanding of what can make you happy. If you're blind, then being able to see would certainly be considered a step closer to a Hotlifestyle, just as getting a restful nights' sleep will also bring you closer to living a Hotlifestyle.

It is time to wake up to the reality that quality sleep is key to your mental and physical wellbeing.

Focus on a structured plan to improve your sleep

It is best to avoid using technology before going to bed, including computers, mobile phones, and television; having a bedtime routine leading up to sleep and calming your mind through 7/11 breathing are simple strategies that make a refreshing sleep more likely. While they may not work immediately, persevere with them each evening. Try to avoid long periods lying down through the day or 'catnapping', even if you're not sleeping soundly at night.

You will sleep for roughly one-third of your life. Sleep in human beings follows a natural pattern called the circadian rhythm. It's a sleep/wake pattern that corresponds to the daylight/darkness cycle.

We also have a natural sleep cycle of about 90 minutes, consisting of five stages.

Understanding the mechanics, identifying the root cause or causes of why you can't sleep then implementing remedies, creating good bedtime habits will get you on the road to success. Time to put on your pyjamas (we'll talk more about that later too) and curl up with a good book - this one will help.

A ruffled mind makes a restless pillow
~ Charlotte Brontë

Sleep is a naturally-occurring, periodic, and recurrent state of unconsciousness which gives the mind and body time to recuperate.

CHAPTER ONE

The Mechanics of Sleep

The Rhythm of Life

It's only recently that scientists have been able to fully understand the alternating cycle of sleep and waking, and how it is related to daylight and darkness. If you are to lay down strategies for a better night's sleep, then there are three important natural patterns you need to understand.

1. Circadian Rhythm

Experiments in the 1700s showed how circadian rhythms worked in plants, causing them to open during the day and close up at night. Humans also have a built-in biological, circadian clock. It's an internal timekeeping device that tells us when to sleep, when to wake, when to eat. It regulates many of our physiological processes over a 24-hour period (circadian comes from the Latin circa, meaning 'around', and dies, meaning 'a day'). There are many examples of circadian rhythms: have noticed that you will tend to wake up at the same time, whether you've set the alarm or not.

The most important gland that exhibits this rhythmic pattern is the pineal gland (located just above the middle of the brain), which is responsible for secreting the hormone serotonin. Serotonin acts as a neurotransmitter that influences brain cells related to mood, sexual desire, appetite, sleep, memory, learning, temperature regulation, and some social behaviour. Levels are highest at noon and lowest at midnight, whereas the secretion of the hormone melatonin (derived from the chemical serotonin) is highest at night and stops in the early hours of the morning. Increased levels of melatonin will make you feel lethargic. This is why early risers find it difficult to sleep in, as their biological clock has already reacted to the wake-up juice, serotonin.

This subject is so important that researchers studying chronobiology (the biology of time and internal biological clocks) were awarded the 2017 Nobel Prize in Physiology for their discoveries of molecular mechanisms controlling the circadian rhythm.

THE CRUX OF IT

The circadian rhythm is our response to light and dark. Routinely going to sleep and waking up at the same time each day helps achieve quality sleep.

2. Sleep Cycle

One full sleep cycle refers to a period of about 90 minutes, during which you progress through five stages of sleep, 1, 2, 3, 4 and REM (rapid eye movement). This means that if you sleep continuously for 7½ hours you experience five full sleep cycles that progress cyclically, then begin again with stage 1 about every 90 minutes. After REM sleep, you return to stage 1 of light sleep and begin a new cycle. Each stage can last somewhere between 5 and 15 minutes.

It is recommended that you achieve
five sleep cycles every 24 hours.

Graph by EL Hartmann MD (The functions of sleep) shows how during eight hours of sleep you might drift into the various stages of sleep.

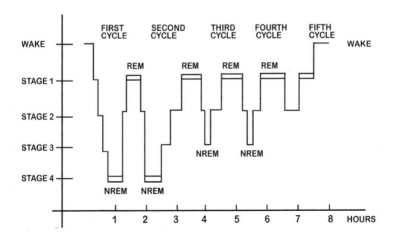

The Five Stages To One Sleep Cycle

Stage 1 (light sleep)

You drift in and out of sleep and can be easily woken. During this stage, you may experience hypnic jerks (sudden muscle contractions) preceded by a sensation of falling. You lose sensory attachment to the physical world toward the end of stage 1.

Stage 2 (light sleep)

Your body temperature begins to drop, and the heart rate slows in preparation for deep sleep. You spend about half your sleep time here in a light dreamless sleep.

Stage 3 (deep sleep)

This is the beginning of deep sleep and another dreamless stage of sleep. It is the period when sleep walking, bed wetting, or talking in your sleep occurs. It's harder to be woken up but should that happen at this stage you will feel especially groggy and confused for a couple of minutes.

Stage 4 (deep sleep)

This is the deepest sleep phase and the most restorative. Not getting enough deep sleep in this phase will leave you feeling groggy in the morning. If roused from this state, you will feel quite disoriented for a while.

REM (REM sleep)

Brain wave activity mimics that of being awake. The eyes move rapidly from side-to-side, hence the name rapid eye movement (REM). It is reckoned that this stage is important for healthy brain function, including the creation of long-term memory. This is the only phase within which you will dream. Should you be woken up during REM phase you can easily slip straight back into this stage when you go back to sleep.

THE CRUX OF IT

View your sleep pattern in blocks of 90-minute sleep cycles. If you sleep for exactly seven hours, you will have woken up in the middle of your fifth sleep cycle, which robs you of your REM phase. It's much healthier to wake up after the cycle is complete and in a light sleep stage.

3. Chronotype

A person's chronotype identifies their sleep preference in a 24-hour period and indicates their most productive time of day. There are two types: morning (early risers, best in the morning), and evening (night owls, best in the evening). This has practical implications for industry, such as morning types should be given morning shifts and evening types evening shifts, which is likely to help increase your performance.

THE CRUX OF IT

Know which chronotype you are. If you're an early riser you might consider going to bed at, say, 10:00 pm, so five sleep cycles of 90 minutes have you getting up at 5:30 am.

Without enough sleep,
we all become tall two-year-olds

~ JoJo Jensen

Sleep Deprivation

The first documented world record holder for sleep deprivation, stayed awake for over 11 days in 1964. At the age of 16, Randy Gardner from San Diego decided to do a school project to see how long he could stay awake without the use of any drugs or caffeine. By the second day he had problems focusing properly and felt fuzzy-headed; by the third day he became moody and angry with his friends. At this stage he was unable to repeat common tongue twisters like 'Peter piper picked a peck of pickled peppers'. On day four he began to hallucinate and by day five he complained of dizziness and his speech began to slur.

As the days passed, Gardner had problems remembering what he said from one minute to the next and the hallucinations grew worse. After completing 11 days and 20 minutes he then slept for 15 hours and seems to have come out of the experience unscathed. At the time of writing this book he is alive and well.

The current world record was achieved in April 1977 and stands at 449 hours (18.7 days). It is held by Maureen Weston, of Cambridgeshire, England.

The category has now been withdrawn due to the inherent risks involved.

Consequences of Sleep Deprivation

The above highlights the short-term consequences of sleep deprivation. Long-term neurological repercussions include loss of motivation, drowsiness, and the inability to make decisions. Studies have also shown that long-term sleep deprivation facilitates weight gain as blood sugar levels can run amok, and it increases blood pressure, depression, and can even cause death. Fatigue, feeling shattered throughout the day, is the most prominent symptom people complain of.

Drowsiness when driving

Sleep deprivation is a daily road safety concern. Drowsiness can slow reaction time as much as driving when drunk. The National Highway Traffic Safety Administration estimates that fatigue is a cause in 100,000 car crashes and 1,550 crash-related deaths each year in the USA. Also bear in mind, if you stop to take a nap try to sleep for one full cycle of 90 minutes to avoid waking up during stages 3 or 4, which will leave you feeling groggy.

Night and day shifts

When your regular routine changes it disrupts your circadian rhythm, which can lead to accidents and injuries at work. In one study, workers who complained of excessive daytime sleepiness were more prone to accidents - and had more sick days.

Jet Lag

Dreading your next long-haul flight? Crossing three or more time zones wreaks havoc with your circadian clock and can result in relentless insomnia, debilitating fatigue, and tormented bowels. There's no way to avoid jet lag, all you can do is alleviate the symptoms by tricking your body clock by planning ahead.

Before you fly

Travelling west: A few days before travelling go to bed one hour later each night and get up later.

Travelling east: Go to bed one hour earlier each night on the three days leading up to your flight.

During the flight

Drink plenty of water. Avoid sleeping pills or alcohol, both of which will hinder your adjustment to the new time zone. Being at high altitude multiplies the effect of alcohol on the body and, since alcohol dehydrates, disturbs your sleep patterns even further. Even one glass will worsen your jet lag symptoms. During the flight set your watch to your destination time and try to eat and sleep on the plane as per that time.

Fasting during the flight

A Harvard Medical School study showed that fasting for at least 16 hours before your arrival can help to override your biological clock. Your digestive system has a lot to do with setting your internal clock. Even if you can't fast, eating as little and as lightly (fresh fruit) as possible can help alleviate some jet lag symptoms.

On arrival

Travelling west: Get outside in the afternoon sun to help shift your circadian rhythm forward. Recovery time is a little less than one day for each time zone you've crossed.

Travelling east: Get more morning sun to help shift your circadian rhythm backward. Recovery time is a little more than one day for each time zone you've crossed. Travelling east causes more severe, longer lasting symptoms.

No matter how tired you are when you arrive, don't sleep more than one cycle during the day. Better still, try to force a new rhythm by going to bed at your normal time, using local time. Try to read rather than watch television. Eat meals at normal set times and try to avoid eating through the night. Especially on your first day, stop eating at 4:00 pm until breakfast the next day. If your journey is shorter than three days, it is worth trying to keep to your home time during the trip.

Insomnia

Insomnia is a sleep disorder characterised by having trouble falling and staying asleep. Lots of factors can contribute to insomnia, so it's not always obvious what the cause is. It can also be accompanied by another health condition, which is why you should consult a physician if you have periods of insomnia for more than three days.

Only go to bed when you're tired. If you haven't fallen asleep within 30 minutes, get up and do something relaxing, like reading (but not on a screen as LED displays glow with blue light, which suppresses melatonin) until you feel tired enough to try again. Don't clock watch, it will only frustrate you even more about being awake and stop you getting to sleep. It is useful to go through bedtime rituals, as described later.

Yoga is an effective bedtime ritual. Just a few yoga poses prior to going to bed can lead to a blissful night's rest.

Learn some yoga poses for better sleep:

hotlifestyle.info/vit/y4s

Cognitive behavioural therapy (CBT) and mindfulness can help you deal with any worries that may be causing sleep problems. CBT helps you to understand what healthy sleep is and how to deal with any negative thoughts about sleep.

Promoting a Good Night's Sleep

Sleep is vital to the recuperation of the subconscious mind and is essential for repairing the body's cells and tissues. Experts at the Harvard Medical School looked at MRI scans of volunteers' brains to see which parts are activated after a good night's rest. They found that sleep helps new memories to 'stick' in the brain - a process scientists call memory consolidation. This happens when connections between brain cells are strengthened by proper rest.

You can find more information on:

 hotlifestyle.info/vit/SAM

Sleep also improves learning capabilities, increases your attention span, and aids in decision making. We've all heard the phrase 'let me sleep on it'. Sleeping on a problem can often result in your creative mind finding a solution. Finally, the processes required for growth and to boost the immune system are also intricately involved with sleep.

Bedtime shouldn't just be when you collapse after a hard day's work. It's the start of an important phase that allows your body and mind to recuperate. You should therefore treat your bedtime with proper respect. No one can dictate your perfect bedtime routine, develop one that feels right for you.

CHAPTER TWO

Sleep Strategies

Move More, Exercise Less

There is a clear connection between poor sleep and a lack of movement. Exercise increases serotonin and dopamine levels, which help to reduce anxiety and depression. However, workouts that last longer than one hour can increase cortisol levels, which might keep you awake, if you exercise in the evenings too close to bedtime.

The UK Department of Health recommends 30 minutes of exercise a day that raises your heart rate slightly, such as brisk walking, dancing, gardening, or climbing stairs. If you're office based, then try to move around at least every 90 minutes.

Resistance exercise, such as lifting weights or body weight exercises, build muscle, while cardio exercise, such as jogging and cycling, work your heart and lungs.

All movement burns calories, even day-to-day activities.

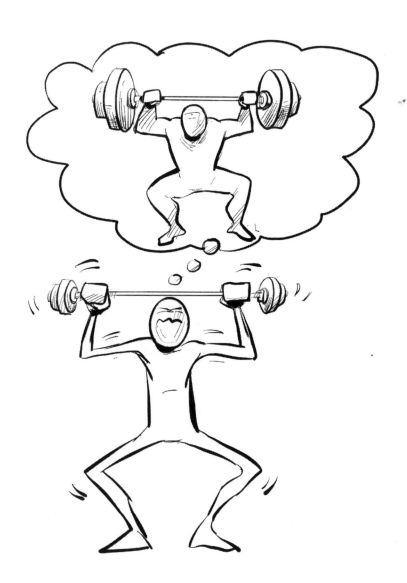

Strategy 1 - Get more movement into your day

➢ **Work at a standing desk** - put your computer on a raised surface so you're standing, which burns more calories than sitting and is better for your posture.

➢ **Use the stairs** rather than taking the lift wherever possible.

➢ **Carry shopping bags by hand** - make sure you have an even load on each side.

➢ **Get a pedometer app** to keep track of your steps and do at least 10,000 a day - pace while on the phone and do short errands on foot rather than driving.

➢ **Clean the house** and put some effort into it, or do some gardening - you'll get fresh air and top up on vitamin D.

➢ **Set a timer** to go off every 90 minutes to remind you to get up and move - a few squats or push-ups all add up over the day.

Avoid taking naps

An obvious thing to avoid, however tempting.

Getting to Sleep

Strategy 2 - Get your sleeping environment right

For half the time in your bedroom you should have your eyes closed - and the rest should be sleeping. That's right, bed is either for sex or sleep!

Make your bedroom a sanctuary - not your office, a TV room or a party room. Create a positive association between your bedroom and sleep by:

➢ making it completely dark, which helps release melatonin

➢ keeping it quiet, with no disruptive beeping of phones

➢ turning your alarm clock so you can't see the time

➢ giving it an optimum room temperature of a cool 16-18 °C (60-65 °F)

➢ using several layers of bedding, so that you can adjust your body temperature if you get too hot or cold

➢ Some suggest sleeping naked

Further reading on choosing the right bed:

 hotlifestyle.info/vit/matt

Strategy 3 - Cultivate a Pre-Bedtime ritual

Stress and anxiety are the main reasons people have difficulty falling asleep Try these techniques to prepare a busy mind for good night sleep:

➢ Try to go to bed at the same time each night - BUT only go to bed when you're feeling sleepy

➢ Use dimmed lights before going to bed in rooms such as kitchen, bathroom and bedroom

➢ Take a relaxing bath about an hour before bedtime - add baking soda and bath salts to warm water

➢ If you opt for a warm shower run it colder at the end

➢ Drink warm milk or camomile tea an hour beforehand

➢ Magnesium helps alleviate night leg cramps

➢ Put a few drops of essential oil of lavender on a tissue and place it under your pillow

➢ Ask your partner for a foot massage

➢ Try the 7/11 breathing method

➢ Capture your inspiration with a daily diary

Learn some great methods to help you get to sleep:

hotlifestyle.info/vit/BM

Staying Asleep

Strategy 4 - Don't be woken up by hunger

If you tend to wake up in the early hours feeling hungry, you could take a light, healthy, low GI snack an hour or two before going to bed. This should not become a regular habit, try to organize your daily eating routine better.

Some light bedtime snack ideas are: 100% whole-grain crackers or bread with a slice of turkey or fatty fish, scrambled egg, handful of walnuts, banana, kiwi, papaya or few sour cherries (like Richmond, Montmorency, or English morello). You could drink sour cherry juice, a camomile or passionflower tea or cup of warm milk with honey. Milk and other dairy products are known sources of tryptophan which is needed to build the sleep hormone melatonin. Milk has been shown to improve sleep in older adults, especially when paired with light exercise.

If you suffer acid reflux you may consider eating 2-3 hours before going to bed to avoid the symptoms. Further reading on:

 hotlifestyle.info/vit/SR

Don't drink large amounts of fluid up to two hours before bedtime and go to the bathroom just before going to bed.

Strategy 5 - Find the right sleeping position

A restful night sleep has much to do with comfort so, forcing yourself to take a certain sleeping position is counterproductive. But not every position that feels good, is actually good for you. Sleeping on your front for example, is one of the worst positions for your health, especially if you have neck or spine issues.

Sleeping on your back with a pillow under your knees not only keeps facial skin free from pillow induced wrinkles, but it also protects your spine and can help relieve hip and knee pain. The best-case scenario for this sleeping position, is not to use a head-pillow at all. If it becomes too uncomfortable, opt for a pillow that is as thin and soft as possible. However, if you tend to snore or are an exceptionally light sleeper, you may find it difficult to rest lying on your back. Then, you will probably feel better lying on your side. Avoid curling up into the foetal position (the most popular), as this can put a huge strain on your back and neck again.

Studies say that right-handed people should sleep on their left-hand side, while lefties will be most comfortable sleeping on their right side. In both cases make sure to choose a good pillow to avoid neck and back pain. A pillow, about 40-centimeter-long and 80-centimeter-wide is for side-sleepers suitable and position another pillow between your knees to keep your hips, pelvis, and spine in better alignment.

Strategy 6 - What you eat matters

A well balanced diet eating natural and nutrient-rich foods and avoiding pollutants and irritants, forms the basis for health and wellbeing promoting a good night sleep. The subject is covered in detail in the next chapter.

Strategy 7 - Have a plan if you are disrupted

Is your partner a different chronotype? You should have asked THAT question on the first date. Living with a night owl when you're a morning person can cause conflict in the relationship. Someone putting on the light or climbing between the sheets when you're asleep, can really disrupt a cycle. With a little consideration the night person could get ready for bed at the same time (after all, bedtime is an important time to connect at the end of the day) as you go to bed, leaving a few minutes later then returning as quietly as possible when they are ready for some shuteye.

If one partner moves around more, consider a bigger bed with a memory foam mattress. It's quite common in Europe that a double bed has two separate mattresses which can be adjusted individually.

Not only do men snore more than women, they also tend to be rowdier. Avoiding alcohol and sleeping on the side may be enough to alleviate snoring. Gently rolling someone on their side can help. If snoring is extreme, then seek professional help to be sure there aren't any underlying health issues. Some couples sleep in separate beds/rooms. Noise pollution is cited as the third most common reason for affecting sleep patterns. Apart from using ear plugs, you can combat noise pollution by playing other background sounds that have a steady soothing effect. It doesn't have to be music, white noise, or the sound of a vacuum cleaner can be just as effective.

If you really can't get back to sleep after being disrupted, don't lie there awake, have a plan. Get up and do some small mundane tasks, like cutting out coupons from magazines ect. Go through your pre-bedtime rituals and avoid putting on bright lights, which will wake you up all the more.

Waking Up in the Mornings

Strategy 8 - Create a Post-Sleep routine

After your fantastic night's sleep, the first 90 minutes of the day are the most important to achieving a good start, so having a morning routine can be really beneficial. Waking up at the same time each day is healthy, as we know, so no sleeping in on weekends. A cool room combined with a warm comfy bed can make the decision to get up difficult. Fortunately, technology has moved on when it comes to alarm clocks. There are clocks that will gradually increase the light in the room before playing music, certainly a much more civilized way to break your slumber. Here is a suggested routine after the clock has gone off.

A Morning Routine

1. While still in bed stretch like a cat.

2. Get up and let plenty of light into the room.

3. Make your bed properly.

4. Some people find taking a daily shower invigorating.

5. Down a full glass of lukewarm water in one go.

6. Have a coffee/tea and breakfast approx. 20 min. later.

7. Set aside at least ten minutes each morning for you.

Start your day with a yoga session:

 hotlifestyle.info/vit/YS

Power up your day with this routine:

 hotlifestyle.info/vit/MR

CHAPTER THREE

Time for a Wake-up Call

WHAT You Eat Matters

Today's fast-paced, consumer-orientated world simply encourages unhealthy lifestyle choices, especially when it comes to food and physical exercise. The statistics speak for themselves. The United States of America has the highest rate of obesity in the world, which means more than 33% of adults are classified as obese. The United Kingdom is not far behind, with around 28% of adults classified as obese. During the past 30 years, obesity has skyrocketed across Western countries. On the other hand, less than 7% of the population of industrialized nations like Japan, India, and China can be considered obese.

Have you ever lied in bed struggling to get to sleep, with your digestion system being anything but quiet? Or have you experienced a restless sleep because you ate too late, and your dinner was still churning in your stomach? Plenty of studies have proven that people who consume foods rich in fat, sugar, protein or too spicy just before going to bed, tend to sleep less deeply and display greater signs of restlessness at night. Fatigue and exhaustion the next morning are inevitable.

To avoid sleep problems, the evening meal should be taken at least two hours before going to bed. If the food is very substantial or heavy, it is advisable to allow at least three hours between dinner and bedtime.

Foods to avoid before bedtime

Too much raw foods in the evening can cause bloating and slow the digestion. Eat fresh, healthy salads at lunch times and steamed, boiled, or fried vegetables in the evening.

Raw fruit, eaten in the evening can't be digested properly before going to bed and can remain fermenting in the intestine. Avoid any raw fruit after 3 pm.

Spicy foods can cause heartburn, flatulence (meteorism) and indigestion making a restful sleep impossible.

Coffee and caffeine rich products (tea, chocolate, energy

drinks...) have a stimulating effect reducing melatonin levels keeping you awake.

A large amount of sugar or carbohydrates (which convert into sugar in the blood) for dinner, not only prevents you from losing weight, but it also leads to problems falling asleep and can even cause a sleepless night as well as producing an even greater craving for sugar the next day.

Alcohol consumed late at night not only disrupts deep sleep but also prevents the body from regenerating. Limit alcohol consumption to one glass in the evening - If you must take a drink, stick with red wine.

How alcohol and marijuana affect sleep

Both substances will have you falling asleep quicker, and both promote a deeper sleep in stages 3 and 4 - good news for insomniacs. However, this is offset by increased sleep disturbances in the second half of the night as the effects wear off. Once alcohol has been metabolized, REM sleep is suppressed, and awakenings are common. Alcoholics report having no dreams because of the disruption of REM sleep.

Studies have shown that long-term use of marijuana leaves you wanting to nap during the day, which suggests a lack of quality sleep. Users report more intense dreams for a while after they stop using.

HOW You Eat Also Matters

There are certain things that can be learned from all that dietary information we are bombarded with - after all, there are genuine reasons why you do lose weight, feel or sleep better if you follow it.

Manage blood sugar levels with foods that have a LOW GLYCAEMIC INDEX (GI) rating, that will make you feel fuller for longer, promoting an improved nights' sleep.

 hotlifestyle.info/GI

Your digestive system breaks down carbohydrates (found in grain, potatoes...) into glucose (sugar), which enters the blood and is utilized for energy by the body. Because of this, foods containing carbohydrates (carbs) can raise blood sugar levels more than other nutrients. Don't confuse this with refined sugars, we are talking about the natural process of your body converting carbs into glucose for energy.

Fibre is also a type of carbohydrate found in vegetables, fruits, nuts, beans, and whole grains which is non-digestible, but makes you full and helps prevent constipation.

The glycaemic index (GI) is a recognized ranking of how different carbohydrates (carbs) will raise blood sugar (glucose) levels when eaten. So, eating high-fibre, low GI foods has been shown to reduce your risk of type 2 diabetes and heart disease, significantly lower cholesterol levels, and promote friendly gut bacteria in the process. Eaten as a snack before bedtime will promote a restful nights' sleep.

Eat fewer grains, potatoes, and sugars - these GPS foods rapidly increase blood glucose levels. High levels of glucose are highly inflammatory and will keep you awake.

Eat a balanced diet. This should be a daily intake of about 60% 'good,' fibre-dense carbs, 25% proteins and 15% healthy unsaturated fats (contained in nuts, seeds, fish, avocado, etc.).

Low calorie, watery, plant-based foods - such as fruit, vegetables, and salads - are bulky, filling and provide key vitamins and minerals.

Fibre fills you up, keeps you full for longer, and can help clean your gut. Great high-fibre foods are: split peas, black beans, kidney beans, chickpeas, lentils, green peas, asparagus, broccoli, Brussels sprouts, cabbage, raspberries, blackberries, avocado, carrots (raw), artichoke hearts, all kinds of nuts...

Protein suppresses your appetite. Eat sources of protein like meat, poultry, fish, eggs, and dairy in moderation. Consumption of red meat preferably lean shoudn't exceed 17oz (480g) a week and fish 7oz (200g) a week. High protein, vegan-friendly, plant-based foods - such as tofu, lentils, edamame, broccoli, spinach, avocado, Brussels sprouts, beans, nuts, and seeds - should be included in your diet more often. For more reading on protein and fibre go to:

 hotlifestyle.info/FP

Eat foods rich in tryptophan. Tryptophan is a naturally occurring essential amino acid found in many foods. To promote a good nights' sleep, your evening meals should include foods containing tryptophan such as, soybeans and soy products, milk and dairy products, eggs, chicken and turkey, fish, avocado, peanuts, pumpkin and sesame seeds, sunflower seeds, and cashew nuts. Tryptophan plays an important role in the production of serotonin, a mood stabilizer, as well as melatonin, which helps regulate sleep patterns.

Tryptophan in supplement form can cause a number of unpleasant side effects like heartburn, headaches, stomach pains, belching, vomiting, nausea, and diarrhoea. Instead of tryptophan supplements, your doctor may recommend 5-HTP supplements instead, which is tryptophan before it's fully converted into serotonin. 5-HTP is not found naturally in any foods that we eat and can also have side effects such as: anxiety, shivering or serious heart issues. Always consult your doctor before taking any supplements that increase serotonin levels especially if you're taking other medications such as antidepressants like SSRIs and MAO inhibitors.

Nutrients That Help Promote Sleep

Vitamin C - insufficient vitamin C intake can lead to depression, which is usually associated with sleep disorders. Vitamin C is vital for the conversion of tryptophan into 5-hydroxytryptophan, the precursor of serotonin.

Magnesium - Helps muscles relax and can trigger a calm, 'sleepy' feeling. Take magnesium glycinate in the evening which is better absorbed than magnesium oxide.

B vitamins - Taking enough vitamins B3, B5, B6, B9, and B12 improves your sleep. They help regulate levels of the amino acid tryptophan. Supplement in the mornings, using a vitamin B complex.

Vitamin D - This 'sunshine vitamin' has also been proven to promote sleep. Dietary sources include fish, beef liver, cheese, and eggs. The UK government has advised everyone to take a 10 mcg vitamin D supplement daily.

Copper - People with copper deficiency have increased adrenaline levels due to decreased excretion. High levels of stimulating adrenaline in the blood causes cardiac arrhythmias, which can also lead to a lack of sleep.

hotlifestyle.info/vit/suppl

Inflammation and the Right Foods

Studies have shown that, there is a clear connection between poor sleep and inflammation. Those who suffer with inflammation tend to spend less time in the REM sleep phase and fail to achieve deep sleep. As I have already said, REM sleep is extremely important for many of the body's functions and crucial for new and long term memories. Endorphins for pain relief and growth hormones for healing are also released during the REM phase. A lack of REM sleep will have negative side effects as your body struggles to regenerate. There are two types of inflammation, 'clinical' and 'sub-clinical.

Clinical inflammation

You hit your knee and your immune system springs into action, it becomes inflamed, painful, and swells up. This is a normal and effective response that facilitates healing.

Sub-Clinical (Chronic) inflammation

Sub-clinical, or chronic inflammation is less obvious since it has no visible signs or symptoms. It is something we ALL have in varying degrees and it can last for months or years if we fail to address the cause. Think of it as an internal irritant that turns on the disease process, causing chronic health issues associated with ageing. It is systemic and affects your organs and internal structures. Chronic inflammation increases the risk of arthritis, heart disease, cancer, diabetes, hypothyroidism, and weight gain. Despite the proven connection between diet and sub-clinical inflammation, doctors don't always consider diet in response to these ailments.

What causes Sub-Clinical inflammation?

Dietary and environmental toxins can build up in the body, turning the immune system on and keeping it highly reactive. A poor diet, stress, a sedentary (couch potato) lifestyle and a lack of sleep all contribute to chronic inflammation.

Researchers believe it is due to an overactive immune system flooding the body with defence cells and hormones that damage tissues. The Western-type diet - high in sugar, fried foods, refined grains (GPS), and high-fat dairy products - promotes high levels of inflammation. Many people still choose convenience over health. Fast foods and convenience foods make up a significant and unhealthy proportion of our diet.

You might compare it to feeding the cat with lettuce. It's the wrong food for the animal. We humans are eating foods containing well known allergens that cause our levels of inflammation to increase.

On the other hand, the Mediterranean diet, green leafy vegetables, and fish, and low in red meat and butter, with moderate alcohol and moderate to high olive oil intake, shows lower levels of inflammation.

Everything in moderation

Foods that promote inflammation are robbing you of your sleep and making you ill. Be aware of them and try to eat less of them. Keep reading, for some fantastic alternatives.

Inflammation-Causing Foods
Grains-Potatoes-Sugars (GPS)

Grains
Avoid milled refined grains (a process that removes the bran and germ to give it a finer texture), such as white bread, white rice, corn flakes, or spaghetti. Whole grains can be eaten in moderation, such as wholewheat bread, buckwheat, oats, millet, brown or wild rice, spelt, amaranth.

Potatoes
Potatoes have a high GI rating, so overeating them can stimulates a big insulin response that, over time, leads to inflammation. Enjoy smaller servings of a lower GI variety (Carisma or Sweet) potatoes, combing them with foods that counteract glucose, like beans and green vegetables.

Sugar and refined starch
Consuming soda, snack bars, candy, baked sweets, sucrose, and lactose leads to a rapid increase in blood sugar; which, in turn, causes insulin levels to rise and triggers an immune response. The result is a pro-inflammatory response leading to chronic inflammation. Avoid anything with added or artificial sweeteners.

One thing most people don't realize is how damaging fructose (fruit sugars) can be, so they should be eaten in moderation. Here is a list of foods containing high levels of fructose:
hotlifestyle.info/FR

Vegetable oil

Found in mayonnaise, salad dressings, barbecue sauce, and potato chips, vegetable oil has high concentrations of the inflammatory fat omega-6. The healthy alternatives are oils rich in omega-3 like olive oil and oils derived from nuts and seeds like chia, flax or hemp. They contain omega-3 fatty acids in the form of alpha-linoleic acid, which helps prevent our immune system from overproducing cytokines and oxidizing molecules that can lead to inflammation.

Dairy products

While moderate amounts of yogurt with gut-healing probiotics help decrease inflammation, full-fat dairy products, soft cheeses, yogurt, butter, ice cream - is a source of inflammation-inducing saturated fats and decreases the levels of our good gut bacteria, which are key players in reducing inflammation.

Red meat

Eating red meat produces a chemical called 'Neu5gc', to which the body produces an inflammatory immune response. Limit red meat consumption to 85 grams a day.

Processed or fast foods? Avoid at all cost!

Don't despair! Everything in moderation.

I can hear you now. "So, what can I eat? No chips, no fast foods, yet another group of foods on the watch list." There are several lifestyle factors contributing to inflammation that are under your control. Learn to relax more, if you smoke then quit, and engage in regular exercise. Diet is only part of the mix. By all means eat your favourite foods just in moderation. Use the Hotlifestyle Healthy Shopping List to guide you. See the link to download a print friendly version of it on the next page.

It's Time for Anti-Inflammatory Diet

Green leafy vegetables
Spinach, kale, romaine lettuce, and Swiss chard are full of natural anti-inflammatory agents and rich in antioxidants.

Cruciferous veggies
Cauliflower, cabbage, garden cress, bok choy, broccoli, Brussels sprouts, celery are high in antioxidants, and all have a natural detoxifying effect.

Fish
Fatty fish, such as wild salmon, mackerel, tuna and sardines, are high in omega-3s.

Nuts
Focus particularly on walnuts (be careful if watching your

weight is an issue and have no more than seven a day), also good are almonds, Brazil nuts, cashews.

Superfoods
Get away from processed foods and replace them with fruit and veggies from your local supermarket. Berries contain lots of fiber and antioxidants such as quercetin, which support the formation of healthy intestinal bacteria and have a preventive effect against diseases of the large intestine. Beetroot contains the antioxidant betalain, which helps repair cells that have been attacked by inflammation. This vegetable also supports blood circulation and contains anti-inflammatory minerals potassium and magnesium.

Download/print the Hotlifestyle Healthy shopping List:

hotlifestyle.info/HD

Probiotics
A large part of the immune system is located in the intestine and is controlled by intestinal bacteria. When the number of harmful microorganisms exceeds the number of beneficial bacteria, a microbial imbalance develops, which increases the risk of inflammation and the risk of many diseases. Probiotic foods such as kimchi (Chinese cabbage), sauerkraut, kombucha, yoghurt or kefir can help harmonize the intestinal flora.

hotlifestyle.info/vit/flora

Detoxification for Quality Sleep

The idea that you can flush your alcohol-drenched liver of impurities and leave your kidneys squeaky clean with a few cups of herbal tea or pills is utter nonsense. There are some unscrupulous marketeers who use the word 'detox' as a pseudo-medical concept to sell something for which there is no evidence that it works. Don't waste your money on so-called 'detox regimes'. You already have a fantastic 'detox' system, if you didn't, you'd be in hospital. Drinking plenty of water, eating healthy and limiting alcohol to a minimum is all the detox you need.

Water water everywhere

A minimum of 1.5 litres of water is required daily just to carry out basic functions like body temperature regulation, transport of nutrients, and removal of waste (detox). We recommend drinking at least 2 litres per day for the average adult living in a temperate climate. This amount ensures your kidneys have enough fluid to flush out harmful toxins

So, the best detox is a large glass (1 pint /0.5 litre) of lukewarm water first thing in the morning the minute you get up. Then wait 20 minutes before you have breakfast.

Be aware of diuretics. Drinks containing alcohol or hot drinks such as tea or coffee increase the need to urinate, making you lose fluids. Plain tap water is always the best option.

CHAPTER FOUR

Anxiety and Sleep

All That 'Self-Talk' Inside Your Head

Anxiety can be triggered when you ask yourself: What might happen? Can I handle it? Do I have what it takes? What if it's not OK? Will it go wrong? Anxiety can also arise from something happening right now that has woken up your fight or flight mode. Anxiety can convert into feelings that have physical effects. During an anxiety attack the physical symptoms become the main issue, overriding what caused the anxiety in the first place.

When you're anxious, your heart rate increases, which then causes your brain to 'race'. An alert mind is far too stimulated to sleep. To make matters worse, an active brain triggers other worries, making it even harder to get to sleep. Once this pattern sets in, bedtime can become an anxious time. So, how can you combat that stress?

Your anxious brain is always on the lookout for possible 'danger'. When there is no real danger out there, your mind takes over and worries, you expect the worst. Physical symptoms may develop, such as panic attacks. The pathway in your brain for anxiety becomes stronger. It can connect your worries with your body's physical symptoms.

Your brain pays attention when you worry about a meeting or dread going somewhere because you might have an anxiety attack. It creates new pathways relating to anxiety. Now while trying to get to sleep you think about the 'meeting' or the place 'you dread going' your anxiety pathway is activated, and your brain starts your anxiety reflex.

You have your own automatic pilot for worries and the physical symptoms can appear automatically. What your brain pays attention to becomes real to you.

 hotlifestyle.info/ST

Practical Anxiety Management

There's no quick fix. You need to commit to making lifestyle changes that promote a more relaxed way of life. With the right tools you can calm your anxiety so that it no longer affects you as much.

Strategy 9 - Calm your anxiety

Exercise releases endorphins, hormones that improve how you feel. Taking up jogging will immediately contribute to your physical and mental health. Studies have compared jogging to taking medication without the side effects.

Eating a healthy diet helps keep your brain and gut healthy, both of which can be linked to your mental health.

Cut out stimulants - the obvious ones are caffeine, ginseng, nicotine and alcohol. Chocolate contains theobromine, which is another stimulant.

Drink water as dehydration worsens the symptoms.

Take supplements such as magnesium, kava, ashwagandha, valerian root, B-complex, St. John's wort, or fish oils.

hotlifestyle.info/vit/sups

Not everybody will react the same to the above ideas. Try them out to find the one that suits you best.

You can manage your heart rate by placing your hand on your heart and listening to the beat. Breathe in deeply for four seconds, and then breathe out slowly. Repeat this and relax, you will feel your heart rate slowing.

Eliminate your anxious thoughts by practising the speaking technique. This means voicing the thoughts that would otherwise live in your head. Speaking aloud overrides thinking, which stops your negative thoughts in their tracks. Think through the alphabet in your head, and when you reach 'G', start speaking out loud. What happened to the alphabet? Well, you stopped thinking it in your head, because speaking overrode those thoughts. Use this technique when you start worrying in bed. Instead of thinking 'the monthly sales figures are down', say aloud 'we will find a way to make the sales this month'.

If anxiety is getting in the way of a good night's sleep, then start working on some anxiety winning strategies.

Breathing for relaxation

Research has shown that how you breathe is intricately connected to your emotional state. You can control your state by changing your breathing pattern. If you breathe in a calm, controlled manner, surrounded by an aroma (real or imagined), savouring each deep slow breath, it has a profound calming effect. Calming natural essential oil fragrances are lavender, camomile, ylang ylang, lemon, yuzu, clary sage, or jasmine.

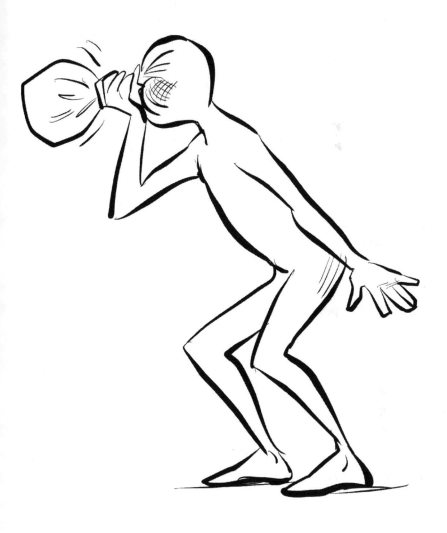

Deep breathing

Sit down with your back straight, place one hand on your stomach. Breathe in slowly from the abdomen and through your nose for a count of 7, fill your lungs with as much air as possible. Breathe so that you feel your lower abdomen rise and fall. Then hold it for a few seconds and breathe out slowly through your mouth, for a count of 11 (breathe out like you're whistling) repeat 10 times.

CO_2 Rebreathing

Erratic breathing, often the result of an anxiety attack can cause hyperventilation, which causes too much oxygen to enter your blood, giving you symptoms like dizziness and a rapid heartbeat. Hold a paper bag over your nose and mouth while you breathe, keep breathing normally to regain your carbon dioxide levels.

7/11 Breathing

Breathing exercises, such as the 7/11 method described over the page, will calm down the nervous system, and the muscles they supply, relaxing tense muscles preventing sudden spasms and keeping you awake.

The 7/11 Breathing Method

1. Take in a deep breath, allow the stomach and lower ribcage to expand as you breathe in.

2. Breathe out, control the flow so that it is steady and slow, empty out a little more than normal (both through the nose, if possible).

3. Continue taking deep breaths in and long, slow breaths out. When you have got used to how it feels, count the length of your breaths.

4. Breathe in for a count of 7 and out for a count of 11.

5. Adjust the speed of your counting so that it is comfortable.

6. The important thing is to make sure that the out breath is longer than the in breath. This triggers an automatic relaxation response in your body.

7. Continue this for 5 to 10 minutes, or however long you wish. Focus on the feeling and the sound of your breathing.

8. As you breathe slowly, be aware of where your body is supported and think of allowing your muscles to let go of the weight of your body on to whatever you are resting upon.

CHAPTER FIVE

Stress and Sleep

When the Pressure's On

The line between stressful and anxious emotions is often blurred because they cause similar symptoms, such as rapid breathing and increased heart rate. The cause of acute stress is plainly different from the cause of anxiety. Stress is the result of how we deal with pressure in our day-to-day lives and you can identify and deal with what is causing it, ‚the trigger'. Anxiety comes from feelings of helplessness and worry that continue after the stressor is gone. The two emotions come from two different places and, despite the differences, many people mistakenly use the terms interchangeably.

Life-threatening situations can cause stress and trigger the ‚fight or flight' instinct in us by releasing adrenalin and cortisol, which give us a burst of energy to help us survive.

Responses to inappropriate levels of pressure

We will all experience pressure in our lives to varying degrees. More pressure means more stress, but what is stressful to one person may not be perceived as stressful to another. What causes you stress depends, in part, on your perceptions and how you cope with the stressors that do affect you. There's a whole list of things that are particularly stressful, like losing your job, getting a divorce, or money problems. The most stressful encounters in life are generally due to unplanned changes in your personal circumstances. Stress is accumulative and often emotionally charged but nowadays not a question of survival.

Long-term stress creates elevated levels of adrenalin and cortisol (known as the stress hormone), which can lead to serious health issues. Many people are unaware that they're suffering from the results of stress and go to the doctor with symptoms of indigestion, back pain, headaches, and so on. The symptoms of stress are broad and not always obvious.

It's important that you become aware of the early warning signs of stress overload, because they can sneak up on you. Very often symptoms become a normal part of your everyday life and are not taken seriously enough.

hotlifestyle.info/stress

Practical Stress Management

Strategy 10 - Beef up your stress tolerance levels

Take responsibility for your life. If you feel that your circumstances are controlling you, and not the other way around then you are more likely to feel overwhelmed. Taking responsibility and controlling your destiny will boost your confidence and alleviate stress.

Take on the challenge and embrace change. Having a positive outlook on life, looking for solutions and not problems is key to reducing stress. Life will throw things your way no matter who you are, it's the way you deal with them that makes the difference. Stop saying, why me?

Create a support network of friends and family. Having reliable people around you to talk with can help with life's pressures. Often, just venting your frustrations can lower stress levels.

Manage your expectations. Having a clear understanding of the mechanics of your stress and how long you can expect it to last, makes it easier to deal with.

Deal with your emotions. If you react emotionally to everything people say to you, learn how to become more emotionally intelligent.

 hotlifestyle.info/life/EQ

If you're suffering from stress, then read the advice given for anxiety - take enough exercise, eat a healthy diet, cut out stimulants, drink at least two litres of water a day, and take supplements.

What Kind of Stress Do You Experience?

In other words, how do you react under pressure? People have different responses to different pressures. Understanding your response is key to deciding how you should deal with it. It is important you learn to relax. I hear you now, 'but I relax every night in front of the telly'. That's good, but it's not going to give you the psychological benefits of deep relaxation. Once you master one of the relaxation techniques, then you will have an 'aha!' moment and understand the difference.

We have already mentioned the fight or flight response, when your brain weighs up the best course of action in a split second, and then you react. What strategy do you tend to choose?

Fight

Do you get angry, aggressive, impatient, shout a lot, or throw things around when you're under pressure? This is typical behaviour from a ‚Type A' personality. You need to quiet down. Deep breathing, progressive muscle relaxation, or meditation would be useful.

Flight

Does pressure make you feel sad or withdrawn, or even give you feelings of being completely spaced out? Which makes you a 'Type B' personality. Try rhythmic exercise (like aerobic training or jogging), power yoga, a massage, or mindfulness. You will probably respond better to activities that stimulate your nervous system as opposed to too much relaxation.

Which Relaxation Technique Suits You Best?

If your stress response is being activated every day, then over time it will take its toll on your emotional health. After all, stress is a natural part of our lives, it's unavoidable. Just as your body has a stress response you also have a natural relaxation response. You've already had your first encounter with a relaxation response when you used the 7/11 deep breathing technique.

When you are in a state of deep relaxation, stress cannot exist. You can balance your body and mind by practising these techniques. When you activate a relaxation response your heart rate will slow, breathing is easier and slower, you become completely relaxed, and your blood pressure normalizes.

Progressive muscle relaxation

This is a technique that creates a relaxation response by tightening and relaxing muscle groups, starting with your feet and working up your body. Tense muscles are one of the side effects of stress and using progressive muscle relaxation allows you to get a feel for the difference between being tense and being relaxed. You need about 15 minutes to complete the exercise.

➢ Remove your shoes and loosen your clothing

➢ Lie down on a mat on the floor or on your bed

➢ Put your hand on your stomach and breathe deeply for 2 minutes from your abdomen so your hand rises and falls

➢ Start by tightly clenching the muscles in your right foot

➢ Focus on the tension built up and hold for 5 seconds

➢ Release the tension and really relax your right foot

➢ Exhale as you release the tension and think the word 'relax'

➢ Imagine your foot sinking into the mat as you relax

➢ Notice the difference between tension and relaxation and repeat this tense/relax action for all the muscle groups in the following order:

1. Right foot - curl your toes downward and hold

2. Right lower leg and foot - pull your toes toward you

3. Entire right leg - squeeze thigh muscles together and hold

4. Repeat with the left leg

5. Right hand - clench your hand in a fist and hold

6. Entire right arm - tighten your biceps by drawing your forearm up toward your shoulder, keep clenching your fist, and hold

7. Repeat with the left arm

8. Buttocks - squeeze your buttocks together and hold

9. Stomach - pull in your stomach and hold

10. Chest - take a deep breath and hold

11. Neck and shoulders - shrug up your shoulders and hold

12. Face - screw up your face and hold

Playing soothing music and using an essential oil fragrance can enhance the experience. Practise this technique twice a day for two weeks. This will embed it into your psyche. As you become practised, you should be able to create a relax response by thinking of your keyword 'relax' (choose any keyword, just keep it the same).

As you get more confident try combining deep breathing with progressive muscle relaxation for additional stress relief.

Rhythmic exercise

You might not think that exercising is relaxing. As mentioned earlier, it may be more beneficial if you have a ‚flight response' to pressure. Rhythmic exercises - rowing, swimming, cycling, walking or jogging - with their repetitive action can have a calming effect. Practice mindfulness while exercising. Notice the rhythmic movements and how your body feels. Focus on the sensations of your feet or hands. Breathe in time with the rhythm of your exercise.

Power yoga

With its dynamic poses and focus on fitness, power yoga is modelled on Ashtanga yoga. It strengthens your body, increases flexibility, and improves posture and balance. You're going to get sweaty so dress appropriately - and don't overdo it. We do not recommend attempting this type of yoga on your own.

Let's Sum Up

You will have noticed that we have not suggested sleeping pills, melatonin or 5-HTP supplements, which should be considered only in conjunction with a health practitioner.

Create a great sleeping environment by making a sanctuary dedicated only to sleep - and sex.

Promote a good night's sleep by eating well and exercising enough throughout the day.

Cultivate pre-bedtime rituals that help you wind down from the day and prepare for a good night's sleep. Dim the lights.

Avoid 'blue light' emanating from computers, TVs etc.

What is your natural rhythm? Know when to go to bed and when to wake up.

Have a strategy ready if you wake up through the night and have difficulty getting back to sleep.

Create a motivating morning routine.

What You Can Achieve

A clear mind and improved physical health and safety.

Improved concentration and not being irritable.

The 30-Day Vitality Challenge

Water
Start each day with a pint/0.5 litre of lukewarm water.
Monitor your drinking to ensure that you drink a minimum of 2 litres/day; consider carrying a 1 litre bottle around with you. Use a filter for drinking tap water.

Refined sugars
Reduce your intake of refined sugar by half.
One spoon instead of two in tea or coffee for example. I find that lactose-free milk is sweeter and use less sugar because of it, besides it being healthier.

Move more
Go the extra mile and walk short distances instead of driving. Use the stairs more and take the lift less.

Stimulants
Cut down stimulants by 20% each on alcohol, tobacco, and coffee/tea.

Stress
Use stress positively to help you perform.
Understand the stress response of others.

Sleep rituals
Go to bed at the same time each night; wake up at the same time too - this includes weekends.

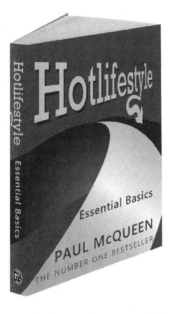

The book you are reading "Sleep Strategies" is a series of excerpts taken from the book **"Hotlifestyle – Essential Basics"** by Paul McQueen.

Essential Basics is 288 action-packed pages helping you achieve goals, become more confident, quelling anxiety and fear of failure, dealing with setbacks, things to help get your life on track. An additional 55 exclusive webpages (videos, tests, further reading) take you deeper into the subject matter leading to a Hotlifestyle. This step-by-step programme is current, relevant, and practical to implement. Presenting the latest evidence-based findings written by experts leading to a healthier happier, richer you.

Essential Basics is a structured no nonsense approach to understanding and dealing with four key areas vital for creating a sustainable difference in your life. The essential basics are; Vitality, Lifeskills, Interactions and Enterprise, each one building on the other.

Achieving a good nights' sleep is obviously an important factor to living a Hotlifestyle. If you're considering changing your job or seeking a new challenge, then Hotlifestyle – Essential Basics will give you a real competitive edge.

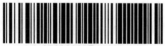